GALLBLADDER DIET

COOKBOOK

Essential Recipes For Digestive Health, Low-Fat Meals, And Friendly Nutrition To Reduce Pain And Promote Healing

DR ELIAN GRIFFIN

DISCLAIMER

The nutritional recommendations and recipes in this book are meant solely for informative reasons. They are not meant to replace the counsel, diagnosis, or care of a qualified medical expert. If you have any doubts about a medical condition or dietary requirements, you should always see your physician or another trained healthcare expert.

All reasonable efforts have been taken by the author and publisher to ensure that the information contained in this book is correct as of the date of publication. Recommendations may alter, though, as medical knowledge is always changing. When using any of the recipes or instructions found here, the user assumes all liability and assumes no risk, whether personal or otherwise. People who have certain dietary requirements or medical issues should speak with a healthcare provider for personalized guidance. The given recipes are only ideas; you may need to adjust them to suit your own nutritional needs, tastes, and tolerances.

When you use this book, you agree to release the publisher, the author, and their representatives from any liability for any claims, damages, liabilities, costs, or expenditures resulting from your use of the book.

TABLE OF CONTENTS

ABOUT THE BOOK

The "Gallbladder Diet Cookbook" is a vital resource for anyone attempting to navigate the complexities of gallbladder health. It is important to realize that a gallbladder-friendly diet has a direct impact on one's overall health, so making dietary adjustments is one way this cookbook helps readers take charge of their health.

This book offers a thorough overview of gallbladder function, common problems, symptoms, and diagnostic insights. It emphasizes how diet plays a crucial role in managing these conditions and preventing their recurrence, emphasizing the impact of nutrition on gallstone formation and overall gallbladder health. Gallbladder issues, ranging from gallstones to more severe conditions, underscore the necessity of dietary modifications.

The gallbladder diet's core principles are outlined in great detail, providing precise instructions on what foods to eat and what to avoid.

A balanced diet, sensible portion sizes, and the importance of water in promoting digestive health are all highlighted. Workable meal plans accommodate a variety of dietary requirements and make meal preparation simple.

Meal preparation tips accommodate busy lifestyles by incorporating efficient kitchen tools to streamline cooking processes. Cooking techniques tailored for gallbladder health promote healthier culinary practices, such as using herbs and spices for flavor enhancement and substituting ingredients for optimal nutritional benefits.

From low-fat smoothies and fiber-rich breakfast bowls to lean protein options and vegetable-based main dishes, the cookbook's extensive recipe collection offers nutrient-rich options that align with gallbladder dietary guidelines. Each recipe is crafted to support digestive health without sacrificing flavor or enjoyment.

The cookbook offers ways to adhere to a diet while traveling and in social situations when it comes to drinks and eating out. Its lifestyle recommendations support overall health and wellness, promoting exercise and stress reduction methods in addition to food changes.

All common issues and frequently asked questions are covered in detail, with helpful advice on how to deal with digestive problems, adjust to dietary changes, and maintain the health of your gallbladder over the long term. It also covers how to handle recurrent symptoms and when to consult a doctor.

"Gallbladder Diet Cookbook" is an indispensable tool for anyone looking to enhance their gallbladder health via dietary control. It does this by fusing nutritional knowledge with useful cooking tips, enabling people to take proactive and long-term control of their health.

CHAPTER ONE

THE VALUE OF A DIET FRIENDLY TO THE GALLBLADDER

For those who have had gallbladder problems or surgery, it is imperative to follow a diet that is friendly to the gallbladder. The gallbladder is an important part of digestion because it stores bile, which aids in the breakdown of fats. If the gallbladder is removed or is not functioning at its best, dietary changes are required to prevent discomfort and aid indigestion. A diet that is friendly to the gallbladder usually emphasizes cutting back on fat intake—especially on saturated and trans fats, which can be more difficult to digest in the absence of bile—and instead emphasizes the consumption of healthy fats like those found in avocados, nuts, and olive oil.

A gallbladder-friendly diet also consists of an abundance of foods high in fiber, such as fruits, vegetables, and whole grains.

Fiber promotes healthy digestion and helps prevent constipation, which can be a problem following gallbladder surgery. It is also important to stay well-hydrated because it helps with digestion and overall health. Foods high in caffeine, alcohol, and spices are often avoided because they can aggravate symptoms like indigestion or abdominal pain in sensitive people. In summary, following a gallbladder-friendly diet promotes digestive health and improves overall well-being by reducing potential discomfort and maximizing nutrient absorption.

Comprehending the fundamentals of a gallbladder-friendly diet enables people to make well-informed dietary decisions that support digestive health. By giving preference to easily digested foods and avoiding those that might cause discomfort, people can effectively manage their diet to promote optimal digestion. This strategy not only aids in adjusting to life without a gallbladder but also enhances overall wellness by guaranteeing adequate nutrient absorption and comfort for the digestive system.

Proactively adopting a gallbladder-friendly diet can considerably improve the quality of life for people who have gallbladder-related issues, cultivating a positive relationship with food, and promoting long-term digestive health.

COMPREHENDING THE HEALTH OF THE GALLBLADDER

Understanding gallbladder health involves recognizing symptoms of gallbladder issues such as abdominal pain, nausea, and bloating, which may indicate the need for dietary adjustments or medical intervention. The gallbladder stores bile, a digestive fluid produced by the liver, which aids in breaking down fats in the small intestine. When the gallbladder becomes inflamed or develops gallstones, it can lead to pain, and digestive discomfort, and possibly require surgical removal.

Genetics, lifestyle, and diet all play a role in gallbladder health. A diet high in cholesterol and saturated fats can increase the risk of gallstone formation, but maintaining a healthy weight and engaging in regular physical activity can lower it.

Gallbladder problems are more common in some groups of people than others, such as women, people over 40, and people with a family history of gallstones. By being aware of these risk factors, people can take preventive measures to support gallbladder health.

THE ADVANTAGES OF A GALLBLADDER DIET

A gallbladder diet has many advantages for digestive health and general well-being. It helps people manage symptoms related to gallbladder problems, like gas, bloating, and discomfort. It does this by emphasizing foods that are easier to digest and minimizing dietary triggers. Lean proteins, healthy fats, and fiber-rich foods are the main components of a gallbladder diet; these foods aid in digestion and support nutrient absorption. It also reduces the risk of digestive distress following gallbladder surgery.

A gallbladder diet also fosters mindful eating practices and a balanced intake of nutrients necessary for general health. It also emphasizes the importance of whole foods like fruits, vegetables, and whole grains, which help people maintain stable blood sugar levels and maintain energy levels throughout the day. It also stresses the importance of adequate hydration to support digestion and remove toxins from the body

HOW YOU CAN USE THIS COOKBOOK TO HELP

This cookbook, which emphasizes low-fat ingredients, lean proteins, and high-fiber foods to promote optimal digestion and nutrient absorption, is a useful tool for anyone looking for advice on implementing a gallbladder-friendly eating plan. It provides a range of recipes that are designed to support digestive health and reduce discomfort related to gallbladder issues or surgery.

Apart from recipes, the cookbook offers helpful advice on meal planning, ingredient substitutions, and portion control, guaranteeing that people can keep a balanced diet without sacrificing flavor or nutritional content. It also informs readers about the fundamentals of a diet that is friendly to gallbladders, enabling them to make decisions about what they eat. Whether dealing with gallbladder problems or recuperating from surgery, this cookbook offers doable fixes and recipe ideas to promote a healthy lifestyle and improve general well-being.

FAST SUCCESS TRICKS

To be successful with a gallbladder diet, realistic tactics must be incorporated into daily routines. Begin by progressively cutting back on high-fat foods and substituting them with healthier options such as lean proteins and plant-based fats. Pay attention to eating smaller, more frequent meals throughout the day to support digestion and avoid overloading the digestive system. Drink lots of water and herbal teas to stay hydrated.

Additionally, prioritize fiber-rich foods like fruits, vegetables, and whole grains to support regular bowel movements and maintain digestive health. Finally, pay attention to your body's cues and adjust your diet as needed to accommodate individual preferences and sensitivities.

CHAPTER TWO

COMPREHENDING GALLBLADDER PROBLEMS

SUMMARY OF KIDNEY FUNCTION

As the little organ beneath the liver, the gallbladder stores the bile that the liver produces, which helps the small intestine break down fats and absorb them into the bloodstream.

When we eat fat-containing meals, the gallbladder contracts and releases bile into the bile ducts, which helps the small intestine break down fats and make them easier to digest—a process that is critical for overall digestive health and nutrient absorption.

Maintaining gallbladder health entails understanding its function and making sure bile production and release are optimized for efficient digestion. Knowing how the gallbladder works is essential to appreciating its role in digestive processes. Without proper bile storage and release, fat digestion becomes inefficient, potentially resulting in digestive discomfort and nutrient deficiencies.

TYPICAL GALLBLADDER ISSUES

Gallstones, which are hardened deposits of bile components that can form in the gallbladder, are one common condition that can affect the function and general health of the gallbladder. Gallstones can vary in size and composition, and some can cause no symptoms at all, while others can cause excruciating pain, particularly if they block bile ducts or cause inflammation (cholecystitis). Other common issues that can affect the gallbladder include bile duct obstruction, gallbladder inflammation (cholecystitis), and even gallbladder cancer, though this is less common.

Early diagnosis and treatment of gallbladder problems depend on the ability to recognize symptoms, which can include fever if inflammation is present, nausea, vomiting, and abdominal pain, especially after eating fatty foods. Diagnostic tests, CT scans, ultrasounds, and blood tests can help healthcare professionals identify the problem and suggest appropriate treatment, which can range from dietary modifications to surgery in extreme cases.

SIGNS AND PROGNOSIS

Abdominal pain, usually in the upper right or middle abdomen, can be the primary symptom of gallbladder problems. Pain can be intermittent or continuous, and it can get worse after eating especially fatty or greasy foods. Other symptoms include bloating, nausea, vomiting, and, in rare cases, fever if there is an infection or inflammation.

The process of diagnosing gallbladder issues usually combines a review of medical history, physical examination, and diagnostic testing; imaging tests, such as ultrasound, are frequently used to visualize the gallbladder and identify gallstones or inflammation; blood tests may reveal elevated liver enzyme levels or infection-related symptoms; and in certain instances, more sophisticated imaging, such as MRI or CT scans, may be required for a thorough diagnosis.

DIET IS IMPORTANT FOR HEALTHY GALLBLADDERS

A healthy balanced diet low in trans fats and high in fiber promotes overall good digestive health; avoiding or minimizing intake of saturated fats, trans fats, and cholesterol-rich foods can lower the risk of gallstone formation; instead, concentrate on consuming healthy fats, such as those found in avocados, nuts, seeds, and fatty fish, which support bile production and digestive processes. Diet plays a critical role in maintaining the health of the gallbladder and preventing complications such as gallstones.

A healthy weight can be maintained and gallbladder problems can be avoided by eating a diet rich in fruits, vegetables, whole grains, and lean proteins. Hydration is also important because it keeps bile fluidity stable and prevents it from becoming too concentrated, which can lead to the formation of gallstones. Physical activity regularly can help manage weight and improve overall digestive function, both of which promote gallbladder health.

Gallstones can be formed or prevented in large part by diet. A diet high in unhealthy fats, and refined sugars and low in fiber can lead to bile imbalances and cholesterol accumulation in the gallbladder, which increases the risk of gallstone development. Conversely, a diet high in fiber, healthy fats, and antioxidants can help maintain bile fluidity and lower cholesterol levels in bile, which reduces the risk of gallstone formation.

A healthy weight through diet and exercise can also lower the risk of gallstones, as obesity is a major risk factor. Drinking enough water throughout the day also supports proper bile function and helps prevent gallstone formation by keeping bile diluted and flowing smoothly. Eating a diet rich in fresh fruits, vegetables, whole grains, and lean proteins is also important for preventing gallstones. These foods also encourage regular bowel movements and help regulate cholesterol levels, which are crucial for gallbladder health.

Knowing how diet affects gallstones allows people to make well-informed dietary decisions that support healthy gallbladder function. People can lower their risk of gallstone development and improve overall digestive wellness by switching to a diet high in nutrients and low in harmful fats.

CHAPTER THREE

THE BASICS OF A DIET FOR GALLBLADDERS

FOOD TO AVOID

Eat a diet high in fiber, such as whole grains, fruits, and vegetables; these foods help control digestion and lower the risk of gallstone formation; healthy fats, such as avocados and olive oil, are beneficial; limit saturated and trans fats, as they can aggravate gallstone problems; and include lean proteins, like fish, chicken, and legumes, as they are easier for the gallbladder to process than fatty meats.

It's also important to avoid some foods. Fried foods, high-fat dairy products, and foods high in cholesterol can all cause gallbladder attacks. Refined sugars, processed foods, and excessive salt should also be avoided to support digestive health in general. You can effectively manage gallbladder issues by eating a balanced diet that emphasizes whole, nutrient-dense foods while avoiding processed and high-fat options.

To maintain the health of your gallbladder and avoid complications, it is important to maintain a balanced diet that includes a variety of carbohydrates, proteins, and fats. Complex carbohydrates, which are found in whole grains and legumes, provide long-lasting energy without taxing the digestive system. Lean proteins, such as those found in beans, chicken, and tofu, are easier to digest and are less likely than fatty meats to cause gallbladder symptoms.

A balanced nutrient intake and an emphasis on whole, unprocessed foods will support optimal gallbladder function and overall well-being. Healthy fats, like those found in nuts, seeds, and avocados, are beneficial for gallbladder function when consumed in moderation. These fats aid in the absorption of fat-soluble vitamins and promote overall digestive health. Additionally, it's important to include plenty of fiber from fruits, vegetables, and whole grains, which support regular bowel movements and helps prevent gallstone formation.

SUGGESTED SERVING SIZES

Aim for smaller, more frequent meals throughout the day to ease the digestive process and prevent gallstone-related symptoms. Incorporate portion sizes that include a balance of carbohydrates, proteins, and fats to support sustained energy levels and digestive comfort. Eating large meals can overwhelm the gallbladder and cause discomfort or attacks.

Planning meals with smaller plates and bowls can help naturally limit portion sizes. You should concentrate on eating foods high in nutrients that supply necessary vitamins and minerals without being overly high in calories or fat. You can better manage gallbladder health and lower your risk of digestive problems by practicing mindful eating and paying attention to portion sizes. Including recommended portion sizes in your daily routine can support overall well-being and promote optimal gallbladder function.

HYDRATION: WHAT IT DOES

Drinking enough water helps prevent gallstones by keeping bile fluid and encouraging regular bowel movements. Aim for at least 8-10 glasses of water per day, adjusting based on individual needs and activity levels. Herbal teas and infused water can also contribute to hydration while offering additional health benefits. Supporting digestion and gallbladder health both depend on adequate water intake.

Apart from water, adding hydrating foods like fruits and vegetables can also help support the gallbladder. These foods are rich in vitamins, minerals, and antioxidants that support digestive health in general.

Avoid consuming too much alcohol and sugary drinks because they can cause dehydration and aggravate gallbladder symptoms. You can support optimal gallbladder function and general wellness by emphasizing hydration with water and hydrating foods.

Individuals can better manage their gallbladder health by creating sample meal plans that are customized to meet their specific needs. For example, if you want to avoid gallstone formation, make sure your meals are low in cholesterol and saturated fats. For breakfast, try oatmeal with fresh berries and a sprinkling of nuts. For lunch, try a quinoa salad with grilled chicken and mixed greens. For dinner, try baked salmon with steamed vegetables and a side of brown rice.

Snack on fresh fruits, nuts, or yogurt throughout the day to maintain energy levels and support digestive comfort. If managing gallbladder symptoms, such as after surgery, choose easily digestible foods that are gentle on the digestive system.

For example, yogurt with sliced bananas and a drizzle of honey could be served for breakfast, vegetable soup with whole grain crackers for lunch, and baked tofu with roasted vegetables, and a small serving of couscous for dinner.

Meal plans should be tailored to each person's dietary preferences and health objectives so that everyone can manage their gallbladder health effectively. People can support optimal digestion and overall well-being by focusing on balanced meals and incorporating a variety of nutrient-dense foods. They can also promote long-term gallbladder health and digestive comfort by adjusting portion sizes and hydration levels as needed to suit individual needs and preferences.

CHAPTER FOUR

COOKING METHODS FOR HEALTHY GALLBLADDERS

HEALTHY COOKING TECHNIQUES

Choosing cooking techniques that minimize the use of added fats and oils—which can exacerbate gallbladder problems—such as baking, steaming, and grilling can help manage symptoms and support overall digestive wellness when it comes to gallbladder health. Baking retains nutrients without using a lot of fat, which makes it perfect for vegetables and lean meats. Steaming keeps food tender while preserving natural flavors and nutrients. Grilling gives meats and vegetables with little to no added fats a delicious charred flavor.

Sautéing with a small amount of heart-healthy oils, such as olive or avocado oil, is another healthy cooking method that enhances flavors and quickly cooks food without overloading the gallbladder with heavy fats. By avoiding deep-frying and choosing these lighter cooking methods, you can also help improve the health of your gallbladder by lowering your intake of fats that can cause inflammation, such as saturated and trans fats.

ADDING SPICES AND HERBS TO FOOD TO IMPROVE FLAVOR

Creative use of herbs and spices can improve flavor in gallbladder-friendly meals while also offering health benefits. Herbs such as parsley, cilantro, and basil add vibrant flavors and freshness to food without adding extra calories or fats; they also contain antioxidants that support overall health and digestion. Spices like turmeric, ginger, and cinnamon have anti-inflammatory properties that can help ease digestive discomfort and soothe the gallbladder.

Increasing the flavor and nutritional value of simple meals can be achieved by experimenting with different combinations of herbs and spices. For instance, a pinch of cinnamon added to oatmeal or yogurt can provide a comforting sweetness without the need for added sugars.

Similarly, fresh herbs can be chopped and sprinkled over salads or added to soups and stews right before serving to enhance their flavor and nutritional value. People who regularly cook with herbs and spices can enjoy satisfying meals that support gallbladder health.

CHANGING INGREDIENTS FOR HEALTHIER ALTERNATIVES

For example, substituting Greek yogurt or low-fat milk for heavy cream in recipes can reduce overall fat content while maintaining a creamy texture. Using lean meats like turkey or chicken breast instead of fatty cuts like beef or pork helps lower saturated fat intake and support digestive health. Substitutions are the key to making gallbladder-friendly meals that are lower in fats, cholesterol, and processed ingredients.

A lighter and more digestible diet can also be achieved by replacing red meat with more plant-based proteins like beans, lentils, and tofu; replacing butter or margarine with unsaturated oils like olive oil or coconut oil can improve heart health and reduce inflammation; and replacing refined flour in baking with whole wheat flour or almond flour adds fiber and nutrients while lowering the glycemic load.

Planning meals ahead of time enables healthier choices and lessens the temptation to choose convenience foods that may be heavy in fats or sugars. Start by selecting recipes that can be easily portioned and stored, such as soups, salads, and stir-fries that contain gallbladder-friendly ingredients. Meal prep is a valuable strategy for maintaining a gallbladder-friendly diet, especially for individuals with busy schedules.

Pre-cutting fruits and vegetables and putting them in grab-and-go containers encourages healthy snacking and meal additions without requiring additional preparation time.

Purchasing high-quality storage containers and labeling meals with preparation dates can expedite the meal prep process and ensure food safety. Batch cooking grains like quinoa or brown rice, as well as proteins like grilled chicken or tofu, provide versatile ingredients that can be quickly assembled into balanced meals throughout the week.

EASY COOKING USING KITCHEN TOOLS THAT ARE GALLBLADDER-FRIENDLY

Having the right tools in the kitchen can make cooking gallbladder-friendly easier and promote healthier food choices. A good food processor or blender can be used to blend nutritious ingredients like roasted vegetables and herbs into smooth soups, sauces, and dips. A steamer basket is a useful tool for quickly preparing vegetables while retaining their nutrients and texture.

Purchasing a nonstick skillet or grill pan can help cut down on the amount of oil used to cook proteins and vegetables, allowing for the use of healthier cooking techniques like sautéing or grilling without sacrificing flavor or texture. Measuring cups and spoons guarantee precise portioning of ingredients, which is critical for a diet that is balanced and supports the health of the gallbladder.

Keeping an assortment of sharp knives and cutting boards on hand can also help with meal preparation efficiency and encourage the use of fresh, whole foods.

People can get the benefits of a diet that is gallbladder-friendly and supports digestive wellness and general health by including these kitchen items in their regular cooking routines.

CHAPTER FIVE

LOW-CARB SHAKES & SMOOTHIES

Smoothies and shakes with minimal fat are great options for a gallbladder diet because they combine nutrition and ease of digestion. They are full of vitamins and minerals and are easy on the stomach. To make a low-fat smoothie, start with a base of almond milk or low-fat yogurt. Then, add your favorite fruits, like mangoes, bananas, or berries, which are high in fiber and antioxidants. You can also add a handful of spinach or kale for extra nutrients without sacrificing flavor. Blend until smooth and enjoy a refreshing drink that promotes gallbladder health.

Shakes can also be prepared with similar ingredients but in different quantities. Choose protein-dense options like whey or plant-based protein powders, which support the maintenance of muscle mass and provide long-lasting energy.

For omega-3 fatty acids, which are good for reducing inflammation, add a tablespoon of ground flaxseeds or chia seeds. Rather than using refined sugars, sweeten your shake naturally with a drizzle of honey or a few dates.

These low-fat smoothies and shakes are not only simple to make, but they can also be tailored to your taste preferences and dietary requirements, which makes them an ideal complement to a gallbladder diet plan.

HEALTHY-FIBER MORNING BOWLS

For optimal digestive health, particularly when following a gallbladder diet, high-fiber breakfast bowls are crucial. Begin by selecting a base that is high in fiber, such as quinoa, bran flakes, or oatmeal; these grains are easy on the stomach and aid indigestion. Next, add a variety of fresh fruits, such as apples, pears, and berries; these fruits are high in soluble fiber, which helps with cholesterol management and fullness.

Finally, to round out the nutritional profile, add a dash of nuts or seeds, like almonds, walnuts, or chia seeds, for additional protein and healthy fats.

These high-fiber breakfast bowls are a great way to get essential nutrients and keep you full and energized throughout the morning. They are simple to make and can be tailored to your taste preferences and dietary restrictions with a variety of toppings. For added flavor and health benefits, try adding a tablespoon of ground flaxseeds or psyllium husk, which are high in fiber and aid in regular bowel movements. Finally, drizzle with a teaspoon of honey or maple syrup for sweetness without exceeding your gallbladder.

TYPES OF OATMEAL AND PORRIDGE

Start by cooking rolled or steel-cut oats with water or low-fat milk until creamy and tender. You can enhance the flavor and nutritional value by adding toppings like fresh fruits like bananas, berries, or sliced apples, which provide vitamins, minerals, and fiber. Oatmeal and porridge are great options for breakfast because they are easy to digest and can be customized with a variety of toppings to suit individual preferences.

These nutrient-dense oatmeal and porridge varieties are versatile and make a great choice for a gallbladder-friendly breakfast that supports digestive health and overall well-being. For extra protein and crunch, sprinkle with a handful of nuts or seeds, such as almonds, walnuts, or chia seeds. You can also stir in a tablespoon of ground flaxseeds or hemp hearts for omega-3 fatty acids, which support heart health and reduce inflammation. Sweeten your oatmeal naturally with a drizzle of honey or a sprinkle of cinnamon instead of refined sugars.

EGG-FREE BREAKFAST SELECTIONS

For people with particular dietary needs or allergies—such as those on a gallbladder diet—egg-free breakfast options are crucial. Thankfully, there are lots of tasty and healthy egg substitutes that can be consumed in different forms. For example, you can make a smoothie bowl in the morning that combines yogurt, blended fruits, and spinach for extra nutrients or you can make a batch of chia seed pudding by soaking chia seeds in almond milk overnight and then topping it with fresh fruit and nuts.

Another great option is avocado toast on whole-grain bread with sliced tomatoes and a dash of sea salt and pepper. Avocados are full of fiber and healthy fats that support digestive health and satiety. If you're feeling particularly cozy, make a bowl of warm quinoa or brown rice porridge with almond milk and top with almonds, seeds, and honey or maple syrup. These egg-free breakfast ideas are not only filling but also simple to make and can be tailored to your dietary requirements and preferences.

IDEAS FOR EASY GRAB-AND-GO BREAKFAST

For a healthy, nutrient-dense, and time-efficient breakfast on a gallbladder diet, try these quick grab-and-go ideas: make overnight oats in a mason jar by mixing rolled oats, almond milk, chia seeds, and a dash of vanilla extract; refrigerate overnight and grab it in the morning for a ready-to-eat, fiber- and nutrient-packed breakfast; or make a batch of homemade granola bars with oats, nuts, seeds, and dried fruits; these can be put in an airtight container for easy on-the-go throughout the week.

For a savory twist, make a batch of veggie-packed mini frittatas using muffin tins and bake until set. These mini frittatas are portable and can be enjoyed hot or cold, making them a versatile choice for busy mornings. These quick grab-and-go breakfast ideas ensure that you start your day with a nutritious meal that supports your gallbladder health without sacrificing taste or convenience. Another convenient option is a whole-grain muffin or breakfast cookie made with ingredients like whole-wheat flour, oats, bananas, and nuts.

OPTIONS FOR LEAN PROTEIN

A diet that is gallbladder-friendly must include lean protein options. Lean proteins are easier for the body to digest and are low in saturated fats, which is good for people who have gallbladder problems. Lean protein options include skinless chicken and turkey, lean beef or pork cuts like sirloin or tenderloin, and fish like salmon, trout, or cod. These proteins are rich in essential nutrients like vitamins B12 and D as well as omega-3 fatty acids, which are important for general health.

Whenever you cook lean proteins, it's best to use low-fat methods such as grilling, baking, steaming, or poaching; these methods preserve flavor without using a lot of oils or butter. You can use seasonings to add flavor without harming your gallbladder; herbs, spices, and citrus juices add zest without adding fat. Eating lean proteins regularly keeps you full and gives you the building blocks you need for muscle growth and repair.

With an emphasis on lean proteins, people can have fulfilling meals that support the health of their gallbladder. These choices aid in digestion and also help people stay at a healthy weight and lower their chance of developing gallstones. Having a wide range of lean protein options makes meal planning flexible and pleasurable while guaranteeing optimal nutrition and comfort for the digestive system.

MAIN COURSES BASED ON VEGETABLES

One of the mainstays of a gallbladder-friendly diet is vegetable-based main dishes, which provide nutrient-dense substitutes for heavier, fattening meals. Vegetables like spinach, bell peppers, zucchini, and mushrooms are high in fiber, vitamins, and minerals, and don't overburden the digestive tract when added to main dishes in inventive ways like stir-fries, vegetable casseroles, or stuffed peppers.

Main dishes made with vegetables are best prepared by roasting or sautéing them to bring out their natural flavors and nutrients.

You can also add herbs, garlic, or low-fat sauces to enhance flavor without compromising the health of your gallbladder. These dishes go well with whole grains or lean protein sources to make well-balanced meals that satiate hunger and ease digestive discomfort.

Vegetable-based main dishes help manage weight and lower the risk of gallstone complications. When prepared mindfully and creatively, vegetable-centric meals become a tasty and beneficial option for people following a gallbladder-friendly diet. A varied range of colorful vegetables guarantees a diverse range of nutrients and antioxidants, which support overall health and well-being.

COMPONENT-BASED SIDE DISHES

Whole grain side dishes are a vital component of a diet for the gallbladder because they supply fiber and vital nutrients while also promoting digestive health. Whole grains such as brown rice, quinoa, whole wheat pasta, and barley are rich in fiber and complex carbohydrates that support sustained energy levels without triggering blood sugar spikes.

Boiling, steaming, or baking whole grains maintains their nutritional value. Adding flavor with herbs, spices, or a light oil drizzle makes them low in fat and cholesterol and a great partner for lean proteins and vegetables. Including whole grains in meals guarantees a diet rich in nutrients and promotes general health and well-being.

Meal planning becomes flexible and pleasurable when a variety of whole-grain options are available. Whole grain side dishes contribute to a balanced diet that helps individuals manage their weight and lowers their risk of gallstone formation. People can enjoy satisfying meals that support gallbladder health and overall well-being by selecting these dishes.

HEALTHY SOUPS AND STEWS FOR THE GALLBLADDER

For those who follow a gallbladder-friendly diet, soups and stews are nourishing and comforting options that support digestive health and provide warmth and moisture. Light yet filling meal options that are easy on the digestive system include broth-based soups with vegetables and lean proteins like chicken or turkey; adding herbs, spices, and a small amount of salt enhances flavor without compromising gallbladder health.

Soups and stews can be made with a variety of vegetables and lean meats, providing flexibility in meal planning while supporting overall wellness. Simmering ingredients slowly allows flavors to blend while maintaining nutrients. Choosing low-fat broth or making homemade broth ensures minimal added fats and sodium, promoting heart health and reducing inflammation.

Soups and stews are a great way to get the necessary nutrients and hydration into a diet for a gallbladder, as well as help with digestion and overall health. Because they are easy on the stomach, they are also a great option for those who are recovering from gallbladder problems or have sensitive stomachs. With easy recipes and healthy ingredients, soups and stews can be a tasty and nutritious part of a well-balanced diet.

PROPERLY MADE SALADS AND DRESSINGS

Salads with the right ingredients and dressings are great options for a diet that is gallbladder-friendly because they are fresh, nutrient-dense, and easy to digest. Leafy greens like spinach, kale, or arugula add fiber and important vitamins that support digestive health and lower the risk of gallstone complications. Colorful veggies like bell peppers, tomatoes, and cucumbers add flavor and nutrients that make salads satisfying and nutrient-dense.

When making salads, wash and chop ingredients well to preserve their freshness and nutritional content. Making your dressings with vinegar, olive oil, citrus juices, and herbs means that there are fewer added sugars and unhealthy fats, which is good for your heart and general health.

You can dress salads with these dressings sparingly to add flavor without overpowering delicate flavors or making you feel queasy.

With a variety of salad combinations and dressing options available, meal planning becomes enjoyable and beneficial while ensuring optimal nutrition and digestive comfort. People can enjoy satisfying meals that support optimal digestion and gallbladder health. These dishes also contribute to a lighter, more digestible diet that may help with weight management.

HEALTHY SNACK SUGGESTIONS

To make your gallbladder diet interesting and fulfilling, try these healthy snack ideas: fresh fruits, such as berries, apples, and citrus fruits, are high in vitamins and antioxidants. These fruits go well with a handful of nuts or seeds for a satisfying crunch and extra protein. Yogurt with honey and granola is another great option; it provides probiotics for gut health and fiber for digestion. For a savory twist, try whole-grain crackers with guacamole or hummus or guacamole.

A balanced snack should contain a combination of carbohydrates, proteins, and fats to sustain your energy levels throughout the day. A few examples of balanced snacks are rice cakes topped with almond butter and banana slices, which provide a combination of complex carbohydrates, healthy fats, and potassium. Vegetable sticks with a light dressing or Greek yogurt dip are also easy and quick options that satisfy your cravings without being heavy or high in saturated fats.

Including wholesome snacks in your daily routine can promote weight management and overall health. If you plan and have healthy options on hand, you can make conscious decisions that promote the health of your gallbladder and your overall well-being. Try a variety of flavors and textures to find snacks that you enjoy and that fit your dietary requirements and preferences.

SIDES OF FRESH FRUIT AND VEGETABLES

A gallbladder-friendly diet must include fresh fruits and vegetables because they are high in fiber and essential nutrients. To optimize the nutritional value of your meals, incorporate a range of colors and textures. To start your day, have a fruit salad or a side of mixed berries for a natural sugar rush and antioxidant boost. For lunch and dinner, have leafy greens like spinach or kale, which are high in vitamins A, C, and K as well as minerals like calcium and iron.

Fresh vegetable sides like cucumber and tomato salad with olive oil and herbs provide hydration and essential fatty acids; these sides support gallbladder health as well as overall digestive wellness and immune function. Vegetables can be enjoyed raw, steamed, or lightly sautéed to preserve their nutrients and natural flavors. Try serving roasted sweet potatoes or squash with a lean protein like grilled chicken or fish for a balanced meal.

To keep things interesting and make sure you're getting enough nutrients, try to have some fresh fruit and vegetables with every meal. You can also add colorful, nutrient-dense sides to your diet by experimenting with different cooking techniques and flavor combinations to find new favorites that work for your palate and dietary requirements.

WHOLESOME SPREADS AND DIPS

Healthy spreads and dips can improve your snacking while promoting a diet that is friendly to your gallbladder. Choose homemade versions that are low in artificial additives and saturated fats. For example, hummus, which is made from chickpeas, tahini, olive oil, and lemon juice, has a creamy texture and plant-based protein.

It pairs well with whole-grain crackers or vegetable sticks for a filling and healthy snack. Avocado, lime juice, tomato, and spices are the ingredients for guacamole, which offers healthy fats and antioxidants.

Greek yogurt-based herb-and-spice-flavored dips are another great option; they provide probiotics for gut health and calcium for strong bones. Try them as a dip for raw veggies or whole-grain pita bread for a well-balanced snack.

Nut butter, like cashew or almond butter, is a great way to get your fill of healthy fats and protein. You can spread them on whole-grain toast or apple slices to add flavor and nutrients that are important for gallbladder health.

Making your dips and spreads at home allows you to be in charge of the ingredients and can tailor the flavors to your tastes. Try different combinations of ingredients and recipes to find new favorites that work well with your gallbladder diet. Including healthy dips and spreads in your daily routine can add flavor and enjoyment to snacking while also promoting overall health and well-being.

MADE-AT-HOME BAKED GOODS

When made with healthy ingredients and in moderation, homemade baked goods can be a wholesome addition to a diet that is gallbladder-friendly. Instead of using refined sugars and excess fats to add sweetness, try using natural sweeteners like honey or maple syrup or whole grains like oats, whole wheat flour, or almond flour as the base for muffins, bread, or cookies. These alternatives offer fiber and important nutrients without compromising taste.

Baking at home gives you control over portion sizes and ingredients, so it's easier to enjoy treats while maintaining the health of your gallbladder. Add ingredients like nuts, seeds, and dried fruits to your baked goods for added texture and nutritional benefits. Chopped almonds or walnuts can enhance muffins or bread with healthy fats and protein. Dried cranberries or raisins can add natural sweetness and antioxidants.

Baking at home can help you create delicious baked goods that satisfy your cravings and support your overall well-being. Just remember to control portion sizes and balance your baked goods with other nutrient-dense foods, and enjoy them as occasional treats rather than daily staples to maintain a balanced diet that supports gallbladder health.

DRINKS: JUICES AND SMOOTHIES FOR SNACKING

Smoothies and juices are nutrient-dense, refreshing snacks that complement a diet that is gallbladder-friendly. To make a base, use frozen or fresh fruits (mango, banana, or berries) for natural sweetness and vitamins; add leafy greens (kale or spinach) for extra fiber, vitamins, and minerals; Greek yogurt or almond milk can add protein and a creamy texture without adding too many sugars or saturated fats; blend until smooth and enjoy as a quick and easy snack.

Add extra omega-3 fatty acids and fiber to your smoothies by adding ingredients like chia, flaxseeds, or hemp seeds.

These seeds can also support gallbladder function and healthy digestion. For a tropical twist, add pineapple juice or coconut water for natural sweetness and hydration. Green juices made with cucumber, celery, spinach, and lemon can also provide you with a boost of nutrients and aid in detoxification.

Smoothies and juices are adaptable snacks that can be tailored to your dietary requirements and taste preferences. Try different fruit, vegetable, and liquid combinations to find flavors that you like. By adding smoothies and juices to your daily routine, you can boost your intake of vital nutrients and promote general health and well-being.

DESSERT RECIPES LOW IN FAT

Desserts like angel food cake, fruit sorbets, or baked fruit crisps are great choices because they are lighter on the gallbladder and also contain vitamins and fiber from fruits that support digestive health. Concentrate on recipes that minimize saturated fats and emphasize healthier alternatives.

For example, you can reduce fat content while adding natural sweetness by substituting butter with unsweetened applesauce or mashed bananas in baking recipes. Look for recipes that use low-fat dairy products like yogurt or skim milk instead of full-fat options.

Try adding whole grains, such as oats or whole wheat flour, to your dessert recipes to increase the amount of fiber and add a nutty flavor. For instance, make oatmeal cookies with less sugar and add dried fruits, such as cranberries or raisins, for sweetness and texture. Cool desserts, such as chia seed puddings or yogurt parfaits with fresh berries, can provide a refreshing treat without sacrificing health benefits. These desserts not only satisfy your sweet tooth but also help you maintain a healthy diet by lowering your intake of fat and promoting overall digestive wellness.

FRUIT-BASED DESSERTS

Desserts made with fruit are a delightful way to indulge in sweets without going overboard with added sugars. To add more flavor and natural sweetness, use seasonal, fresh fruits; fruit salads with a range of colorful fruits, such as melons, berries, and citrus fruits, can be a refreshing and nutrient-dense option; or try grilling fruits, such as pineapple or peaches, and serving them with a drizzle of honey or a sprinkle of cinnamon. These desserts are not only delicious but also a great way to support overall health, including digestive function.

For a more decadent option, consider making fruit tarts with a crust made of whole wheat or almond flour and filling it with a mixture of Greek yogurt and fresh fruit.

These tarts are satisfyingly sweet and provide a good balance of flavors while being gentle on the digestive system. Another option is to make homemade fruit popsicles using pureed fruits and a small amount of honey or agave syrup as a natural sweetener. These frozen treats are perfect for hot days and provide a guilt-free indulgence with minimal impact on your gallbladder.

LIGHTER VERSIONS OF DECLUSIVE TREATS

Sweets can still be included in a gallbladder-friendly diet if you make small changes to the ingredients. For instance, you can make avocado chocolate mousse, which is a creamy dessert rich in antioxidants and healthy fats, by blending ripe avocados with cocoa powder and a natural sweetener like maple syrup or dates. You can also make banana ice cream by freezing ripe bananas and blending them until smooth, then flavoring them with cocoa powder or vanilla extract.

For those who like to bake, try cutting the amount of sugar in recipes by using low-calorie, minimally-affecting alternatives like erythritol or stevia; swap out refined flours for gluten-free almond or coconut flour, which adds a nutty flavor and increases fiber content; desserts like flourless nut butter cookies or coconut macaroons can be decadent, guilt-free treats that are satisfyingly delicious and easy on the gallbladder. With these modifications, you can still enjoy your favorite sweets without sacrificing flavor or health objectives.

BAKING ADVICE FOR DESSERTS THAT WON'T HURT YOUR GALLBLADDER

Baking desserts that are gallbladder-friendly should emphasize cooking techniques that reduce the amount of added fats and oils. Baking or steaming fruits can release natural sugars and improve flavors without the need for additional sweeteners. For example, baking apples with a cinnamon and honey drizzle can result in a warm, cozy dessert that is both nourishing and filling. Use spices like nutmeg or ginger in your baking recipes to add flavor depth without using too many fats or sugars.

Instead of adding salt to recipes, try enhancing flavors with herbs like mint, basil, or citrus zest. These ingredients not only add freshness but also balance out the sweetness of fruits naturally found in desserts. If you're baking cakes or muffins, look for recipes that use mashed bananas or applesauce as binders instead of butter or oil. This will help you consume less saturated fat while maintaining the moist and flavorful texture of baked goods. These baking tips will help you enjoy delicious desserts that are easy on your gallbladder and promote overall digestive health.

TIPS FOR MODERATION AND PORTION CONTROL

Desserts can be enjoyed while adhering to a gallbladder-friendly diet as long as portion control is maintained. To visually manage portion sizes and avoid overindulging, serve desserts in smaller plates or bowls. When indulging in richer desserts, like cheesecake or chocolate cake, cut smaller slices to satisfy your sweet tooth without consuming excessive fats or sugars. When eating dessert, concentrate on savoring each bite and eating mindfully to appreciate the flavors and textures of your dessert.

Desserts can be enjoyed in moderation by limiting them to occasional treats rather than daily indulgences. This helps maintain a balanced diet that supports digestive wellness and overall health. By incorporating these portion control and moderation tips into your eating habits, you can enjoy desserts responsibly while managing your intake of gallbladder-friendly desserts. You can also enjoy social occasions while managing your intake of desserts by sharing them with friends or family.

BOOSTERS OF HYDRATION

Drinking enough water is essential for gallbladder health, but there are other ways to increase fluid intake in addition to plain water. Infused water is a good example of this; fresh fruits, such as cucumber, berries, or citrus slices, can be added to water to naturally flavor it without adding sugar or artificial sweeteners. This is a fun way to stay hydrated, and the vitamins and antioxidants in the fruit help to slightly boost your body's nutritional value.

In addition, coconut water—which is a natural option for people who want to stay away from sugary drinks and replenish vital minerals lost due to dehydration—is another hydration booster. Its electrolyte content supports overall digestive health and helps maintain hydration levels. Herbal teas, like peppermint or chamomile, are also a good option for hydration goals because they are caffeine-free and soothing.

When people choose these hydration boosters over plain water, they can maintain optimal levels of hydration while supporting the health of their gallbladder with extra nutrients and digestive benefits. Regular fluid consumption and urine color monitoring are key components of an effective gallbladder diet.

HERBAL TEAS TO AID WITH DIGESTION

Herbal teas are an important part of maintaining digestive health, especially for those on a gallbladder diet. Peppermint tea, for example, has long been known to relieve gas and bloating as well as other digestive discomforts. It also contains menthol, which helps relax the muscles in the digestive tract, promoting easier digestion and possibly reducing discomfort related to gallbladders.

Another effective option is ginger tea; its anti-inflammatory qualities may help reduce inflammation linked to gallbladder problems; it promotes bile flow, aiding in digestion and possibly lowering the risk of gallstone formation; regular drinking of ginger tea can enhance overall digestive health and is a useful addition to a diet plan for gallbladders.

If you're looking for something tastier, chamomile tea is calming and easy on the stomach. It also helps reduce inflammation in the digestive system and eases stress-related digestive problems. By adding these herbal teas to regular water intake, people can improve their digestive health and enjoy tasty, healthy drinks that go well with a diet that supports the gallbladder.

BLENDS OF FRESH JUICE

Juice blends made with ingredients that support digestive health and reduce potential triggers for gallbladder discomfort are a great way to increase nutrient intake while following a gallbladder-friendly diet. Beetroot, carrot, and apple juice is a popular blend that offers a mix of vitamins, minerals, and antioxidants without overwhelming the digestive system.

Orange and lemon juices, for example, can also be helpful because they contain vitamin C, which boosts immunity and helps with detoxification. It's best to drink these juices sparingly and dilute them with water to lessen their acidity and make them easier on the stomach.

Leafy green juices—like spinach or kale mixed with cucumber and celery—provide a nutrient-dense, high-fiber, and nutrient-rich option that supports overall gallbladder health, regular digestion, and the provision of necessary vitamins and minerals. Through trial and error with various juice combinations and recipe modifications based on individual preferences, people can savor a range of fresh juices that support their dietary goals.

STEER CLEAR OF HIGH-SUGAR DRINKS

It is important to avoid sugary sodas, energy drinks, and commercially processed fruit juices that often contain added sugars and artificial sweeteners. These beverages can cause weight gain and metabolic disturbances, which may aggravate gallbladder-related discomfort.

High-sugar beverages can exacerbate symptoms associated with gallbladder issues, such as blood sugar spikes and increased risk of inflammation.

Alternatively, go for naturally sweetened options such as infused water, homemade fruit smoothies, or herbal teas. These options support stable blood sugar levels and overall digestive health by providing hydration without the negative effects of added sugars. People can make informed decisions that support their gallbladder diet goals by carefully reading labels and selecting beverages that have minimal or no added sugar.

ALCOHOLIC DRINKS SAFE FOR THE GALLBLADDER

Drinking alcohol while following a gallbladder diet means that you have to be mindful of how it affects your digestion and general health. Clear spirits, such as vodka or gin, have fewer congeners (fermentation byproducts that aggravate symptoms), so mix these with water or soda water and flavor with a squeeze of fresh citrus juice. Red wine can also be enjoyed in moderation for its potential cardiovascular benefits, but be aware of its acidity and potential to trigger reflux. Dark liquors, beer, and sugary mixed drinks should be avoided as these can aggravate gallbladder symptoms. By selecting gallbladder-safe alcoholic beverages in moderation and being aware of their ingredients, you can occasionally enjoy a drink while adhering to your dietary goals.

CHAPTER SIX

HANDLING SOCIAL EVENTS AND EATING OUT

GETTING AROUND RESTAURANT MENUS

It's important to know your dietary preferences and limitations when navigating restaurant menus and following a gallbladder diet. Look for lean protein sources like grilled chicken or fish, and choose side dishes like steamed vegetables or a simple salad with vinaigrette dressing. Steer clear of creamy sauces, buttery dishes, and anything that is fried or greasy as these can exacerbate gallbladder symptoms.

You can enjoy dining out while adhering to your gallbladder diet without feeling restricted if you are proactive and knowledgeable about the preparation of the food. Many restaurants are accommodating to dietary needs and can offer substitutions or adjustments to suit your requirements. It's also helpful to check the restaurant's menu online, if available, to get an idea of what options might be suitable before arriving.

While attending social events can be difficult for someone on a gallbladder diet, it is possible to manage these situations with a little planning and strategy. To start, try eating a small, balanced meal or snack before the event to help reduce hunger and avoid overindulging in foods that can aggravate gallbladder symptoms. Once at the event, concentrate on socializing rather than just the food by participating in activities and conversations that will divert your attention from temptations.

If there are self-serve or buffet-style options, take your time to look over all the options before filling your plate; choose lighter options like salads, grilled meats, and vegetable dishes. If possible, let the host know in advance about your dietary restrictions so they can make accommodations for you. Offer to bring a dish that satisfies your diet requirements to share, making sure there's at least one option you know you can enjoy.

Maintaining your gallbladder diet when dining out or at social gatherings requires effective communication with hosts and servers. Begin by letting them know about your dietary needs and preferences; explain that you must avoid certain foods that are fried, high in fat, or highly processed because these can aggravate gallbladder symptoms. Most hosts and servers are understanding and will make accommodations for dietary needs if they are told ahead of time.

Be specific about what you can and cannot eat to avoid any misunderstandings. If you're unsure about a particular dish or ingredient, don't hesitate to ask for more information or recommendations from the server. By keeping open and clear communication, you can enjoy your meal while adhering to your gallbladder diet without feeling uncomfortable or deprived. Ask questions about how dishes are prepared and request modifications if necessary, such as dressing on the side, grilled instead of fried, or substitutions for high-fat ingredients.

TRAVELING AND STILL EATING THE RIGHT FOOD

When traveling on a gallbladder diet, it is necessary to plan and make sure you have access to accommodations and foods that meet your dietary requirements. Before your trip, look up restaurants and grocery stores that will provide options that fit your diet. Bring easy-to-carry, diet-compliant snacks like nuts, seeds, and low-fat crackers so you won't have to rely solely on unfamiliar food options while traveling.

When booking a flight, ask for a special meal that satisfies your dietary needs. This will guarantee that you have a suitable meal when you travel. When dining out, apply the same tactics you would at home: choose grilled or steamed foods, steer clear of creamy sauces or fried foods, and ask for adjustments if necessary. Staying hydrated is also crucial, so bring a reusable water bottle with you and drink lots of water to support your overall health and digestive system.

On a gallbladder diet, managing cravings and temptations requires preparation and mindful awareness to prevent triggers that may cause discomfort. Begin by identifying your particular trigger foods, such as fried snacks, high-fat desserts, or rich sauces, and devise strategies to resist them. When cravings arise, take a break and engage in something else to divert your attention from food, such as taking a walk, deep breathing, or taking up a hobby.

To satisfy cravings without sacrificing your diet, always have healthy snacks on hand at home or on the go. Go for low-fat, high-fiber snacks like whole-grain crackers, fresh fruits, or veggies with hummus. When faced with situations where tempting foods are available, practice mindful eating by enjoying small portions or, when feasible, selecting healthier options. Moderation is the key to managing gallbladder symptoms and preserving general health.

CHAPTR SEVEN

LIFESTYLE SUGGESTIONS FOR HEALTHY GALLBLADDERS

INCLUDING PHYSICAL EXERCISE

Beyond diet and lifestyle modifications, physical activity is essential for overall health. Regular exercise helps prevent gallstones by supporting weight management, but it also improves digestion and overall metabolic health. Start with moderate aerobic exercises, such as brisk walking, cycling, or swimming, for at least half an hour most days of the week. These activities improve blood circulation and reduce inflammation, which can indirectly benefit gallbladder function.

Strength training exercises can help you gain muscle mass and improve your metabolism. Exercises like bodyweight resistance exercises, such as squats and push-ups, can help you improve your overall fitness level and support your gallbladder health journey. If you're new to exercise or have any health concerns, start slowly and see a fitness professional. By incorporating physical activity into your daily routine, you can dramatically improve your overall well-being and gallbladder health.

TECHNIQUES FOR STRESS MANAGEMENT

The health of your gallbladder can be adversely affected by chronic stress, so it's important to learn effective stress management techniques. Deep breathing exercises, yoga, and mindfulness meditation are some of the techniques that can help lower stress levels and promote relaxation. Deep breathing is a technique that you can use to help reduce stress because it triggers the body's relaxation response, which can help reduce symptoms related to stress.

Incorporating regular mindfulness exercises into your daily routine can also improve your capacity to manage stress. Mindfulness is a technique that involves focusing on the present moment without passing judgment, which can help lower anxiety and promote emotional well-being.

You can cultivate a sense of calm and resilience by dedicating a short period each day to meditation or mindfulness exercises. By implementing these stress management techniques into your life, you can support the health of your gallbladder and improve your overall quality of life.

MONITORING YOUR DEVELOPMENT

It's critical to track your progress on the gallbladder health journey to stay motivated and make well-informed decisions. Maintain a journal in which you record your meals, noting foods that cause discomfort or digestive issues, and track your physical activity to make sure you're meeting your goals. You can also use the journal to identify patterns and make necessary lifestyle adjustments.

By tracking your progress systematically, you can optimize your gallbladder health journey and make long-lasting lifestyle changes for long-term well-being. Apart from journaling, you should also think about using technology, such as wearable fitness trackers or apps, to monitor your daily steps, heart rate, and sleep patterns. These tools can offer valuable insights into your overall health and help you stay accountable to your goals. Regularly review your progress and celebrate your achievements, no matter how small.

ASKING FOR LOVED ONES' SUPPORT

It is important to seek support from loved ones when navigating dietary and lifestyle changes. You can get encouragement and motivation by sharing your goals and challenges with friends, family, or a support group. Having a support system can help you stay consistent and overcome setbacks on your path to gallbladder health.

In addition, having open communication with loved ones about your health goals can help them understand how best to support you, whether that be with practical assistance, emotional support, or just being there to listen. Support from loved ones can boost your confidence and commitment to improving your gallbladder health.

You can ask them to join you in healthy activities like cooking nutritious meals together, going for walks, or taking exercise classes. Their involvement can make the process more enjoyable and reinforce positive habits.

WHEN TO SEEK ADVICE FROM A MEDICAL PROFESSIONAL

Effective management of gallbladder health requires knowing when to seek professional guidance. If you experience persistent symptoms like severe abdominal pain, nausea, vomiting, or jaundice, you should seek medical attention as soon as possible. These symptoms may indicate gallbladder disease or other underlying health issues that need to be evaluated and treated by a professional.

A healthcare provider can offer personalized advice based on your unique health status and assist you in creating a customized plan for improving gallbladder health. Regular check-ups and screenings are also crucial for monitoring your gallbladder health and identifying any potential issues early.

By seeking timely medical advice and guidance, you can ensure proactive management of your gallbladder health and overall well-being. Furthermore, you should speak with a healthcare provider before making significant changes to your diet or exercise routine, especially if you have pre-existing medical conditions or are taking medications.

CHAPTER EIGHT

HANDLING DIGESTIVE PROBLEMS

Starting with a diet that is easy on the digestive system is essential when managing digestive problems associated with gallbladder conditions. This usually means emphasizing low-fat, high-fiber foods while steering clear of fried, greasy, and highly processed foods that can exacerbate symptoms. Foods that are easy on the stomach and support regular bowel movements, such as oatmeal, bananas, and steamed vegetables. Drinking lots of water and eating smaller, more frequent meals instead of larger, heavier ones can also greatly reduce discomfort associated with digestion.

Probiotics can also be added to your diet; foods like kefir, yogurt, and fermented foods like kimchi or sauerkraut can help balance the good bacteria in your gut, improving digestion and minimizing bloating. You should also steer clear of foods that are known to aggravate symptoms, like alcohol, caffeine, and spicy foods; keeping a food journal can help you identify and eliminate these triggers, enabling you to customize your diet to your unique needs and lessen the frequency and severity of digestive problems.

A balanced diet and supplement regimen, along with regular, gentle exercise, can greatly improve your digestive health and overall well-being. For those who still have digestive issues, you might want to think about adding digestive enzymes. These supplements can help break down food more efficiently, easing the workload on the digestive system. Always consult with a healthcare professional before starting any new supplement regimen to ensure it's appropriate for your condition.

ADAPTING TO MODIFICATIONS IN DIET

After gallbladder removal, adjusting to new dietary restrictions can be difficult, but with a few doable steps, it can be manageable. First, start by progressively adding low-fat foods to your meals, like lean proteins, whole grains, and an abundance of fruits and vegetables. This helps your body get used to processing food differently without the gallbladder. It's also important to stay away from foods high in fat and cholesterol, as these can be hard for your body to digest without a gallbladder.

Meal planning can be a useful tool to help you follow your new dietary guidelines. By organizing your meals in advance, you can include a range of nutrients while limiting fat content. You can try different cooking techniques, such as baking, grilling, or steaming, which preserve flavor without adding extra fat. You can also maintain a balanced diet by including healthy fats, like those found in avocados, nuts, and olive oil, in moderation. Ultimately, this method not only makes your meals more enjoyable but also supports your digestive system over time.

Maintaining a food journal to document the effects of various foods on your body can provide insightful information and assist you in making educated decisions. Gradually, these modifications can become second nature, making your new diet both sustainable and pleasurable. Eating slowly and chewing food thoroughly can aid in digestion, reducing the workload on your stomach and intestines.

MAKING SURE THERE IS ENOUGH NUTRIENT

A wide variety of nutrient-dense foods, such as leafy greens, lean proteins, and a variety of fruits and vegetables, is excellent choices. These foods are rich in essential vitamins and minerals, helping to support your body's needs without overwhelming your digestive system. It's also beneficial to include foods high in fiber, such as whole grains and legumes, to promote healthy digestion and prevent constipation. Ensuring nutrient sufficiency after gallbladder removal is essential for maintaining overall health and preventing deficiencies.

If you find it difficult to get enough nutrients from your diet alone, you may want to think about adding supplements. A multivitamin can help fill in any gaps, particularly when it comes to fat-soluble vitamins like

A, D, E, and K, which are absorbed with the aid of bile from the gallbladder. Before beginning any new supplement regimen, speak with a healthcare professional to find out what's best for your individual needs.

They can help you create a customized supplement plan that supports your nutrient intake while taking into account any potential interactions with medications or other health conditions.

Furthermore, adding omega-3 fatty acids from sources like flaxseed or fish oil can help with heart and brain health. Eating foods high in these fats, like walnuts, chia seeds, and salmon, can assist you in keeping your intake of essential fatty acids in balance.

Eating a well-balanced diet that provides enough nutrients not only helps you heal but also improves your quality of life by giving your body everything it needs to function at its best without a gallbladder.

Aim for at least 30 minutes of moderate exercise most days of the week. Activities like walking, cycling, or swimming can help maintain a healthy weight, reduce the risk of gallstones, and improve overall digestive health.

Regular exercise also enhances the function of your digestive system, aiding in the efficient processing of food. These are just a few of the lifestyle habits that support digestive health prevent complications and help maintain long-term gallbladder health.

Incorporating a variety of fruits, vegetables, and whole grains into your meals and limiting your intake of processed foods, sugary snacks, and high-fat items are important ways to maintain a healthy weight and lower your risk of gallbladder issues. Drinking plenty of water throughout the day can also aid in digestion and help prevent constipation, which is especially important after gallbladder removal.

In addition to providing advice on how to maintain a balanced diet, control your weight, and address any ongoing digestive issues, routine check-ups with your healthcare provider are crucial for monitoring your gallbladder health and general well-being. Being proactive and knowledgeable about your health can greatly improve your quality of life and prevent complications related to gallbladder health.

HANDLING SYMPTOM RECURRENCE

After having your gallbladder removed, you may find it difficult to manage and alleviate recurrent symptoms. One strategy that may help is to keep a detailed food diary, which can help you identify specific triggers that exacerbate your symptoms and modify your diet accordingly. Common culprits include fatty foods, dairy products, and caffeine. Once you have identified your triggers, you can work towards reducing or eliminating them from your diet.

Adding stress-reduction strategies to your diet, such as yoga, meditation, or deep-breathing exercises, can help reduce symptoms in addition to dietary modifications. Regular physical activity, as previously mentioned, not only supports weight management but also improves mood and overall well-being, reduces stress, and improves digestion. Staying active and involved in activities you enjoy can make a big difference in your symptom management.

Working closely with healthcare professionals can provide you with the support and resources needed to manage recurrent symptoms effectively, ensuring a better quality of life after gallbladder removal. If symptoms persist despite these adjustments, consulting with a gastroenterologist or a dietitian specializing in digestive health may be necessary. They can offer tailored advice and may suggest treatments or medications to help manage symptoms. Additionally, some people find relief through probiotics or specific supplements that support digestive health.